THE COMPLETE SMOOTHIES FOR LUPUS

EASY AND DELICIOUS SMOOTHIES TO SOOTHE INFLAMMATION

KAREN EDMONDS

TABLE OF CONTENT

INTRODUCTION 7

CHAPTER 1 9

Understanding lupus and dietary considerations.......................................9

Benefits of Smoothies for Lupus Patients 12

CHAPTER 2 17

Building blocks of a lupus-friendly smoothie 17

CHAPTER 3 21

Common Ingredients for Lupus-Friendly Smoothies..21

CHAPTER 4: SMOOTHIE RECIPES FOR LUPUS 27

Berry Blast Anti-Inflammatory Smoothie 27

Green Goddess Lupus Warrior Smoothie 32

Tropical Turmeric Bliss Smoothie........37

Nutty Protein Power Smoothie 42

Customizable Smoothie Bowl for Lupus 47

Berry Citrus Immunity Booster 52

Minty Pineapple Green Smoothie 56

Chocolate Banana Almond Bliss 60

Tropical Turmeric Mango Smoothie 64

Protein-Packed Berry Almond Smoothie 69

Spinach Blueberry Bliss Smoothie 73

Creamy Oatmeal Smoothie 78

Apple cinnamon delight 83

Creamy carrot ginger smoothie 88

Kale pineapple refresher 93

Cherry Almond Bliss Smoothie 98

Banana walnut smoothie 103

Creamy Avocado Spinach 108

CHAPTER 5 113

Tips for Preparing Lupus-Friendly Smoothies 113

Fresh vs. Frozen Ingredients 117

CHAPTER 6: CONCLUSION 123

STAY HEALTHY

INTRODUCTION

Individuals living with lupus encounter unique issues that go beyond the scope of conventional care. The quest to manage an autoimmune disorder involves a comprehensive strategy, with diet playing a critical part. Imagine a bright morning full of optimism, when Karen, a lupus warrior, found peace in the simple act of making a nutritious smoothie. Her narrative mirrors the sentiments of many people negotiating the complexities of lupus.

Lupus, a chronic autoimmune illness, appears differently in each person, causing a wide range of symptoms from joint discomfort to skin rash. Understanding the critical link between diet and lupus care reveals an effective tool-the lupus-friendly smoothie. This introduction takes you on a journey through the healing power of combining healthy ingredients, sharing stories of success and perseverance.

The trip goes beyond a simple combination of fruits and greens; it is a story about recovering control, drinking on energy, and enjoying the flavours of sustenance. As we dig into the world of lupus smoothies, we discover a carefully curated list of components designed to treat inflammation, improve energy, and promote overall wellness. Join us as we investigate the transformational power of these elixirs, constructing a tale of health, hope, and a beautiful fusion of nature's wealth and the lupus experience.

CHAPTER 1

Understanding lupus and dietary considerations

Lupus is a chronic autoimmune illness that causes the immune system to assault healthy tissues and organs. It can affect several sections of the body, causing symptoms including joint pain, skin rashes, exhaustion, and organ inflammation. Lupus has no cure, although it is commonly managed with drugs, lifestyle changes, and dietary concerns.

Lupus can affect several systems in the body, including the skin, joints, kidneys, heart, lungs, and brain. Lupus' inflammatory reaction can cause long-term discomfort, oedema, and organ damage. Understanding how lupus affects different organs is critical for making dietary decisions that promote overall health and manage individual symptoms.

Dietary Guidelines for Lupus persons:

A well-balanced and nutrient-rich diet is beneficial for persons with this condition. While there is no one-size-fits-all strategy, typical recommendations include eating a mix of fruits and vegetables, whole grains, lean meats, and healthy fats. Limiting processed foods, salt, and sugar can help manage inflammation and improve general health.

Important Nutrients for Lupus Management:

Lupus symptoms can be effectively managed with specific nutrients. Omega-3 fatty acids, such as those found in fish and flaxseeds, are anti-inflammatory. Vitamin D is necessary for bone health, which is an issue for lupus patients who are frequently on long-term corticosteroid medication. Colourful fruits and vegetables contain antioxidants, which can help neutralise free radicals and decrease oxidative stress.

Hydration and Kidney Health:

Proper hydration is essential for kidney function, as lupus can have an impact on them. Lupus sufferers should drink enough of fluids to help their kidneys function properly. Water-rich meals and beverages, such as smoothies with hydrating components, help to maintain overall hydration.

Balancing Protein Intake: Protein is necessary for tissue repair and immunological function. Lupus patients may develop muscular atrophy or weakness, thus appropriate protein intake is critical. Individual dietary constraints can be accommodated by incorporating lean protein sources such as poultry, fish, tofu, and lentils into the diet.

Calcium and Bone Health:

Certain lupus drugs, notably corticosteroids, might affect bone density. Incorporating calcium-rich foods, such as dairy or fortified plant-based alternatives, promotes bone health. Furthermore, vitamin D increases calcium absorption and is critical for lupus sufferers.

Monitoring Trigger meals: While there is no globally recognised lupus diet, people may discover particular meals that worsen symptoms. Keeping a food diary and consulting with a healthcare practitioner or nutritionist can help you identify and manage possible trigger foods.

Understanding lupus and its effects on the body is critical for making dietary choices that help control symptoms and promote overall health. Lupus patients should collaborate with healthcare specialists and nutritionists to develop a personalised dietary plan that addresses their individual needs.

Benefits of Smoothies for Lupus Patients

Smoothies are a simple method for lupus sufferers to get critical nutrients without stressing their digestive system. Blending fruits, vegetables, and other components breaks down cell walls, allowing the body to better absorb essential vitamins and minerals.

Proper hydration is critical for people with lupus, as it might harm their kidneys. Smoothies, which are commonly composed with hydrating components such as water-rich fruits and vegetables, help to maintain proper fluid levels, improve renal function, and promote overall hydration.

Managing Inflammation: Lupus causes chronic inflammation, which can be exacerbated or alleviated by particular diets. Smoothies may be customised with anti-inflammatory components like turmeric, ginger, and leafy greens, which assist to modify the immune response and decrease inflammation.

Nutrient-Rich Boost: Lupus patients may have nutritional deficits owing to drug side effects or malabsorption. Smoothies include a high concentration of nutrients such as antioxidants, vitamins, and minerals, which promote general health and help to repair any shortages.

Weight Management: Certain lupus drugs may cause weight swings. Smoothies may be a nutritious and customisable weight-management solution. Incorporating healthy fats, protein, and fibre helps to create tasty and balanced smoothies that promote weight stability.

Convenience and time-efficiency: Lupus can cause weariness and joint discomfort, making meal preparation tough. Smoothies are a quick and easy option that need little work to create while giving a high dosage of nourishment.

Customisation for Dietary Preferences: Lupus patients' dietary requirements may vary. Smoothies may be customised to meet specific dietary needs, including dairy-free, gluten-free, and vegetarian alternatives.

Boosting Energy: Lupus-related tiredness is a prevalent issue. Smoothies including fruits, leafy greens, and protein sources can give a natural energy boost, allowing people to manage their daily tasks more effectively.

Improved Gut Health: Lupus sufferers may have gastrointestinal difficulties. Smoothies made with probiotic-rich components like yoghurt or kefir, as well as fibre from fruits and vegetables, help to maintain a healthy gut microbiota, which may alleviate stomach pain.

Improved Medication Compliance: Some lupus drugs are most effective when taken with meals. Smoothies are a tasty and readily digested approach to absorb critical nutrients while taking medicine, enabling improved compliance with specified treatment programmes.

STAY HAPPY

CHAPTER 2

Building blocks of a lupus-friendly smoothie

- ***Anti-Inflammatory Ingredients:***

Incorporating anti-inflammatory substances can help control lupus inflammation. Tumeric, ginger, and green tea are among examples. These substances can help to reduce inflammation and boost overall immunological health.

- ***Nutrient-Rich Fruits:***

Choose fruits with high vitamin, mineral, and antioxidant content. Berries, especially blueberries and strawberries, are strong in antioxidants and can help battle the oxidative stress linked with lupus. Furthermore, citrus fruits such as oranges and grapefruits include vitamin C, which aids in immunological function.

- ***Healthy Fats:***

Consuming healthy fats can improve brain function and decrease inflammation. Avocado, flaxseed, chia seeds, and nut butters are all wonderful options. These fats also add to the smoothie's creamy mouthfeel.

- ***Protein Sources for Lupus Patients:***

Protein Sources for Lupus Patients: Lupus patients may develop muscular weakness or wasting, thus protein consumption is crucial for muscle health. To meet total protein requirements, use protein sources such as Greek yoghurt, tofu, or protein powder (explore plant-based alternatives).

- ***Leafy Greens:***

Leafy greens, like spinach and kale, are high in vitamins, minerals, and antioxidants. They are also high in fibre, which helps with digestion. If you are sensitive to raw greens, simply boiling or blanching them before blending might help them digest more easily.

- ***Dairy-Free Milk Alternatives:***

For lupus patients with dietary limitations, dairy-free milk substitutes such as almond, coconut, or oat milk might serve as a basis. These options give the smoothie a liquid consistency while addressing lactose intolerance and other sensitivity.

- ***Supplements:***

Consider using lupus-specific vitamins or supporting components. Omega-3 fatty acid supplements, vitamin D, and probiotics may be useful. When using supplements, use caution and contact with a healthcare practitioner to establish the proper dosage.

- ***Low-Glycemic Sweeteners:***

To sweeten the smoothie, use low-glycemic sweeteners such as honey, maple syrup, or agave nectar. These options deliver sweetness without generating sudden rises in blood sugar levels.

- ***Hydrating Elements:***

Include hydrating ingredients in your smoothie, such as coconut water or water-rich fruits like watermelon and cucumber. Proper hydration is critical for lupus patients, particularly if renal function is compromised.

- ***Taste and Texture customization:***

Customise smoothies based on personal taste and texture preferences. Experiment with various component combinations to get the ideal balance. Adding frozen fruits or ice can thicken the smoothie and make it more pleasant.

Lupus patients may make tasty and nutritious smoothies by carefully mixing these building blocks, which suit their unique nutritional demands while also contributing to general health and well-being. Always speak with a healthcare practitioner or a trained nutritionist to ensure that dietary choices are appropriate for your specific health needs.

CHAPTER 3

Common Ingredients for Lupus-Friendly Smoothies

Berries:

Blueberries, strawberries, raspberries, and blackberries are high in antioxidants, which help fight inflammation and oxidative stress caused by lupus.

Leafy greens:

Spinach and kale include vital vitamins, minerals, and fibre. For individuals who are sensitive, lightly heating or blanching greens might improve their digestibility.

Turmeric:

Turmeric is known for its anti-inflammatory qualities, and it includes curcumin, which may aid in inflammation management and immunological function.

Ginger:

Ginger contains anti-inflammatory and antioxidant effects. It provides a tangy flavour to smoothies and might aid with digestion.

Avocado:

The avocado adds healthful fats and a creamy texture to the smoothie. It contains monounsaturated fats, which are beneficial to heart health.

Flaxseeds:

Flaxseeds are high in omega-3 fatty acids, making them a plant-based source of these vital lipids, which can help decrease inflammation.

Chia Seed:

Chia seeds are rich in omega-3 fatty acids, fibre, and protein. They give smoothies a gelatinous texture and contribute to a sense of fullness.

Protein sources:

Greek yoghurt, tofu, or plant-based protein powder can be used to improve muscular health, especially if lupus symptoms include muscle weakness.

Dairy-free Milk Alternatives:

Almond milk, coconut milk, or oat milk serve as the smoothie's liquid foundation. Choose dairy-free choices if you have lactose sensitivity or dietary limitations.

Citrus fruits:

Oranges, grapefruits, and lemons may provide a delightful citrus flavour. These fruits include vitamin C, which promotes immunological function.

Coconut Water:

Coconut water is a hydrating basis for smoothies that contains electrolytes and has a somewhat sweet flavour.

Honey or maple syrup:

These natural sweeteners can be used sparingly to give sweetness while avoiding abrupt blood sugar increases.

Cucumber:

Cucumber gives a pleasant aspect and helps with hydration owing to its high water content.

Watermelon:

Watermelon not only hydrates but also provides natural sweetness and a luscious texture to the smoothie.

Cinnamon:

Cinnamon has a warm, sweet flavour and may include anti-inflammatory qualities.

Probiotic-Rich Yoghurt:

For people who do not have dairy allergies, probiotic-rich yoghurt promotes gut health and digestion.

Iced or frozen fruits:

Ice cubes or frozen fruits can increase the thickness and chill effect of the smoothie.

Combining these basic ingredients creates a number of delectable and healthy lupus smoothie choices. Lupus patients should tailor recipes to their specific preferences and dietary limitations.

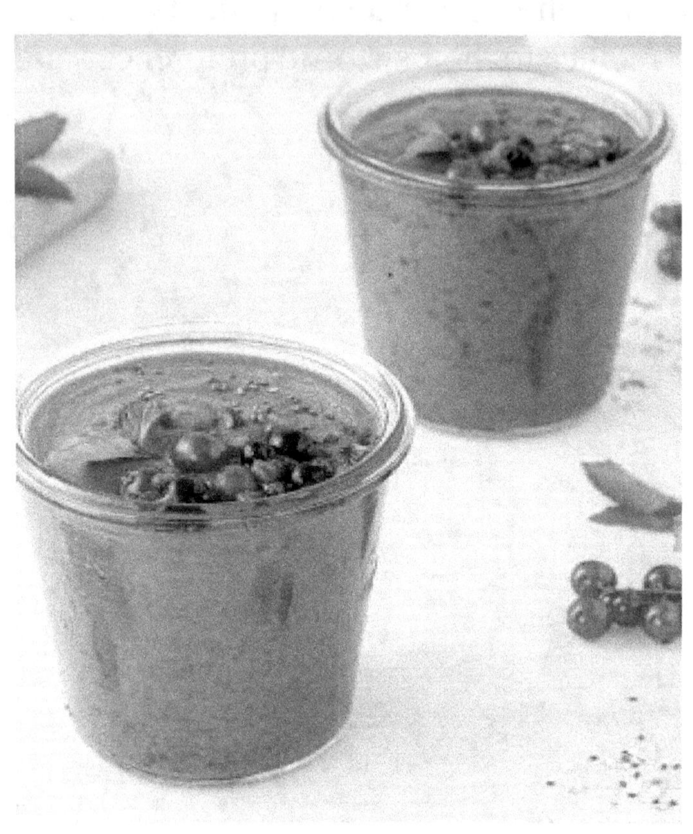

CHAPTER 4: SMOOTHIE RECIPES FOR LUPUS

Berry Blast Anti-Inflammatory Smoothie

Ingredients:

- 1 cup of mixed berries (blueberries, strawberries, raspberries)
- 1/2 cup of spinach leaves (fresh)
- 1/2 teaspoon of turmeric powder or a small piece of fresh turmeric
- 1/2 teaspoon grated ginger
- 1/4 avocado
- 1 tablespoon of flaxseeds
- 1 tablespoon of chia seeds
- 1/2 cup of Greek yogurt (or dairy-free alternative for those with lactose intolerance)
- 1 cup of coconut water or almond milk

- 1 tablespoon of honey or maple syrup (optional, for sweetness)
- Ice cubes (optional)

Instructions:

Get ready the Ingredients:

- Wash the berries and spinach well.
- Peel and cut the avocado.
- Grate some fresh ginger.

Combine the ingredients in the blender:

- In a blender, combine the mixed berries, fresh spinach, turmeric powder (or fresh turmeric), grated ginger, avocado, flaxseeds, chia seeds, Greek yoghurt (or dairy-free substitute), and coconut water (or almond milk).

Blend until smooth:

- Blend all of the ingredients until they are smooth and creamy. If the smoothie is too thick, add additional coconut water or almond milk until you get the required consistency.

Taste and sweeten (optional):

- Taste the smoothie and, if needed, add honey or maple syrup for sweetness. Blend again to include the sweetness.

Serve and enjoy:

- Pour some Berry Blast Anti-Inflammatory Smoothie into a glass.
- If you want, add ice cubes for a colder drink.

Garnish (optional):

- Garnish with a few fresh berries or chia seeds for extra texture and visual appeal.

Sip and get the benefits:

- Sip on this colourful smoothie and enjoy the explosion of flavours while benefiting from the anti-inflammatory effects of berries, turmeric, and other healthy ingredients.

Nutritional Value Per Serving (Approximate):

Calories: 250 kcal

Protein: 10g

Carbohydrates: 30g

Dietary Fiber: 8g

Sugars: 15g

Fat: 12g

Cholesterol: 10mg (when using Greek yogurt)

Sodium: 150mg

Potassium: 600mg

Vitamin A: 50% DV

Vitamin C: 70% DV

Calcium: 20% DV

Iron: 10% DV

Notes

Your

Observation

Green Goddess Lupus Warrior Smoothie

Ingredients:

- 1 cup of kale, stems removed
- 1/2 cup of cucumber, peeled and chopped
- 1/2 ripe banana
- 1/2 avocado
- 1/2 green apple, cored and sliced
- 1 tablespoon of fresh lemon juice
- 1 teaspoon of chia seeds
- 1 teaspoon of spirulina powder
- 1/2 cup of coconut water or almond milk
- Ice cubes (optional)

Instructions:

Get ready the Ingredients:

- Wash the kale well and remove the stems.
- Peel and chop the cucumber.
- Peel and slice a banana.

- Chop the avocado and green apple.

Combine the ingredients in the blender:

- Combine kale, cucumber, banana, avocado, green apple, fresh lemon juice, chia seeds, spirulina powder, and coconut water (or almond milk) in a blender.

Blend until smooth:

- Blend all of the ingredients until the smoothie has a creamy smoothness. If needed, add more coconut water or almond milk to get the desired thickness.

Taste and adjust:

- Taste the smoothie and adjust the flavour as needed by adding extra lemon juice.

Ice cubes (optional):

- If you want a cooler smoothie, add a handful of ice cubes and mix until smooth.

Pour and enjoy:

- Pour some Green Goddess Lupus Warrior Smoothie into a glass.

Garnish (optional):

- To enhance visual appeal, garnish with a piece of cucumber or a sprinkling of chia seeds.

Sip, Feel the Power:

- Drink this nutrient-dense smoothie, incorporating the deliciousness of greens, fruits, and superfoods like spirulina to boost your body and support your lupus journey.

Nutritional Value Per Serving (Approximate):

Calories: 220 kcal

Protein: 6g

Carbohydrates: 28g

Dietary Fiber: 8g

Sugars: 12g

Fat: 12g

Sodium: 60mg

Potassium: 800mg

Vitamin A: 150% DV

Vitamin C: 80% DV

Calcium: 15% DV

Iron: 20% DV

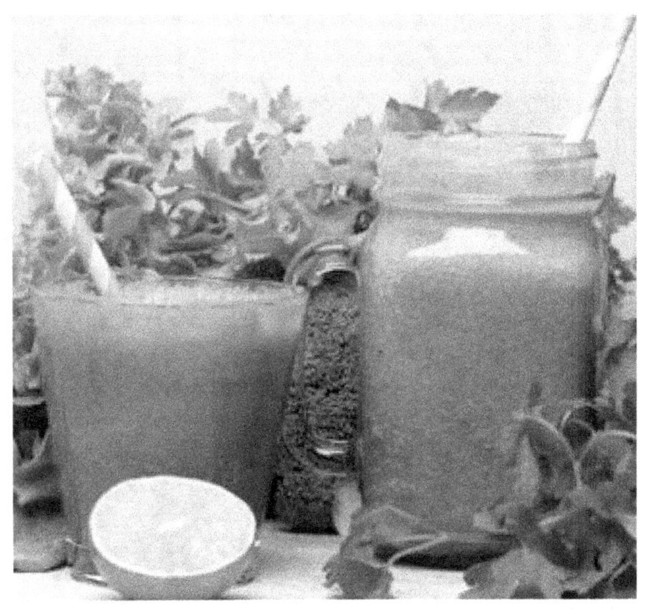

Notes

Your

Observation

Tropical Turmeric Bliss Smoothie

Ingredients:

- 1 cup of pineapple chunks (fresh or frozen)
- 1/2 cup of mango chunks (fresh or frozen)
- 1/2 banana
- 1/2 teaspoon of turmeric powder or a small piece of fresh turmeric
- 1/2 teaspoon grated ginger(fresh)
- 1 tablespoon of chia seeds
- 1/2 cup of coconut milk
- 1/2 cup of fresh orange juice (squeezed if possible)
- Ice cubes (optional)

Instructions:

Get ready the Ingredients:

- If using fresh fruits, peel and cut the pineapple and mango.
- Peel a banana.

- Grate some fresh ginger.

Combine the ingredients in the blender:

- Combine the pineapple, mango, banana, turmeric powder (or fresh turmeric), grated ginger, chia seeds, coconut milk, and orange juice in a blender

Blend until smooth:

- Blend all of the ingredients until they're smooth and creamy. To modify the thickness, add additional coconut milk or orange juice.

Taste and adjust:

- Taste the smoothie and modify the flavour as needed by adding additional ginger or a splash of orange juice.

Ice cubes (optional):

- If you want a cooler smoothie, add a handful of ice cubes and mix until smooth.

Pour and garnish (optional):

- Pour the Tropical Turmeric Bliss Smoothie into a glass.
- To add a tropical touch, garnish with a piece of pineapple or chia seeds.

Sip and Enjoy the Bliss:

- Sip on this Tropical Turmeric Bliss Smoothie and enjoy the tropical flavours while benefiting from turmeric's anti-inflammatory effects and the nutritional value of the fruits.

Nutritional Value Per Serving (Approximate):

Calories: 220 kcal

Protein: 4g

Carbohydrates: 45g

Dietary Fiber: 8g

Sugars: 30g

Fat: 6g

Sodium: 15mg

Potassium: 600mg

Vitamin A: 30% DV

Vitamin C: 160% DV

Calcium: 10% DV

Iron: 10% DV

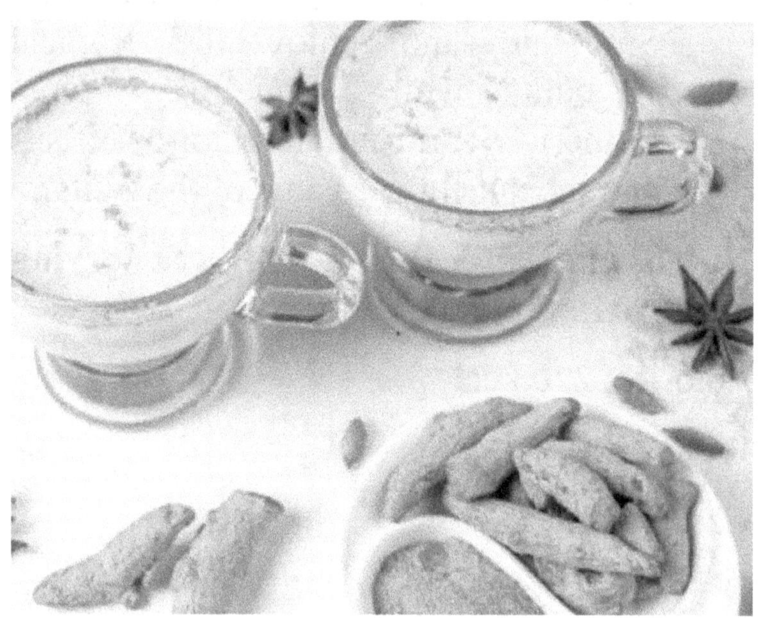

Notes

Your

Observation

Nutty Protein Power Smoothie

Ingredients:

- 1 banana
- 2 tablespoons of almond butter
- 1/4 cup of Greek yogurt (or dairy-free option)
- 1 tablespoon of chia seeds
- 1 scoop plant-based protein powder like Pea protein powder (or any other that is lupus-friendly)
- 1/2 teaspoon of cinnamon
- 1/2 teaspoon of honey or maple syrup (optional, for sweetness)
- 1 cup of almond milk
- Ice cubes (optional)

Instructions:

Get ready the Ingredients:

- Peel a banana.
- Measure out the almond butter, Greek yoghurt, chia seeds, plant-based protein powder, cinnamon, and almond milk.

Combine the ingredients in the blender:

- Combine the banana, almond butter, Greek yoghurt, chia seeds, plant-based protein powder, cinnamon, and almond milk in a blender.

Blend until smooth:

- Blend all of the ingredients until the smoothie has a creamy smoothness. If required, add additional almond milk to get the desired thickness.

Taste and sweeten (optional):

- Taste the smoothie and, if needed, add honey or maple syrup for sweetness. Blend again to include the sweetness.

Ice cubes (optional):

- If you want a cooler smoothie, add a few ice cubes and mix until smooth.

Pour and garnish (optional):

- Pour Nutty Protein Power Smoothie into a glass.

- For extra texture, garnish with chia seeds or almond butter.

Sip & Power Up:

- Sip this Nutty Protein Power Smoothie and enjoy the creamy texture and nutty flavours that deliver a protein boost for long-lasting energy.

Nutritional Value Per Serving (Approximate):

Calories: 350 kcal

Protein: 20g

Carbohydrates: 30g

Dietary Fiber: 7g

Sugars: 12g

Fat: 18g

Sodium: 200mg

Potassium: 600mg

Vitamin A: 2% DV

Vitamin C: 10% DV

Calcium: 40% DV

Iron: 10% DV

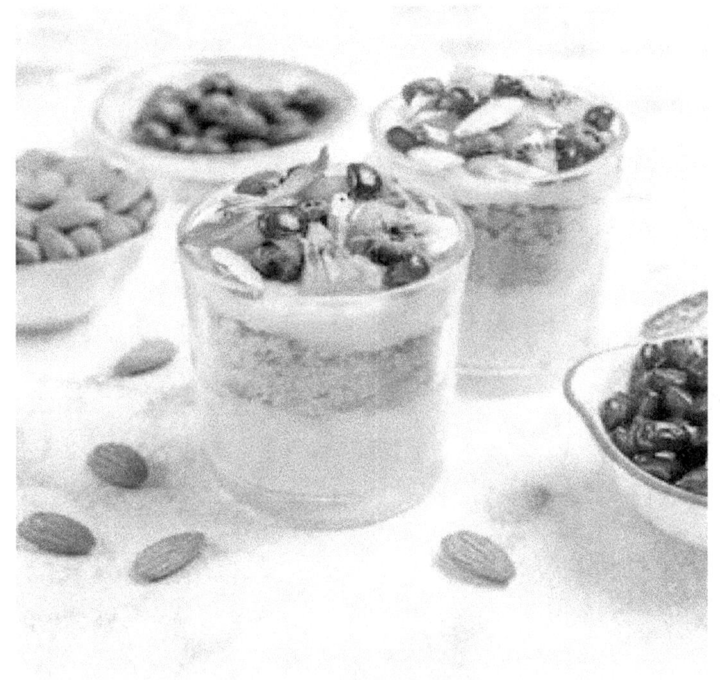

Notes

Your

Observation

Customizable Smoothie Bowl for Lupus

Ingredients:

Base:

- 1 frozen banana
- 1/2 cup of mixed berries (blueberries, strawberries, raspberries)
- 1/2 cup of fresh spinach leaves
- 1/2 cup of Greek yogurt (or dairy-free alternative)
- 1 tablespoon of chia seeds
- 1/2 cup of almond milk

Toppings (select as preferred):

- Sliced fresh fruits (kiwi, mango, pineapple)
- Granola
- Nuts (almonds, walnuts)
- Seeds (pumpkin seeds, sunflower seeds)
- Shredded coconut

- Drizzle of honey or maple syrup (optional)

Instructions:

Get ready the Ingredients:

- Peel and slice the banana.
- If using fresh fruits as toppings, wash, peel, and slice them.
- Measure out the Greek yoghurt, chia seeds, almond milk, and toppings.

Blend the base:

- Add frozen bananas, mixed berries, spinach, Greek yoghurt, chia seeds, and almond milk in a blender
- Blend until you get a smooth, thick consistency.

Customise your bowl:

- Transfer the smoothie base to a bowl.
- Arrange your desired toppings on the smoothie base. This is where you may get creative by selecting a range of textures and flavours.

Drizzle (optional):

- If you want to add sweetness, sprinkle honey or maple syrup over the toppings.

Enjoy your customisable smoothie bowl:

- Grab a spoon and enjoy your personalised smoothie bowl, savouring the combination of flavours and textures.

Nutritional Value (Approximate):

Calories: 350 kcal

Protein: 15g

Carbohydrates: 50g

Dietary Fiber: 12g

Sugars: 25g

Fat: 12g

Cholesterol: 10mg (when using Greek yogurt)

Sodium: 100mg

Potassium: 800mg

Vitamin A: 80% DV

Vitamin C: 70% DV

Calcium: 40% DV

Iron: 15% DV

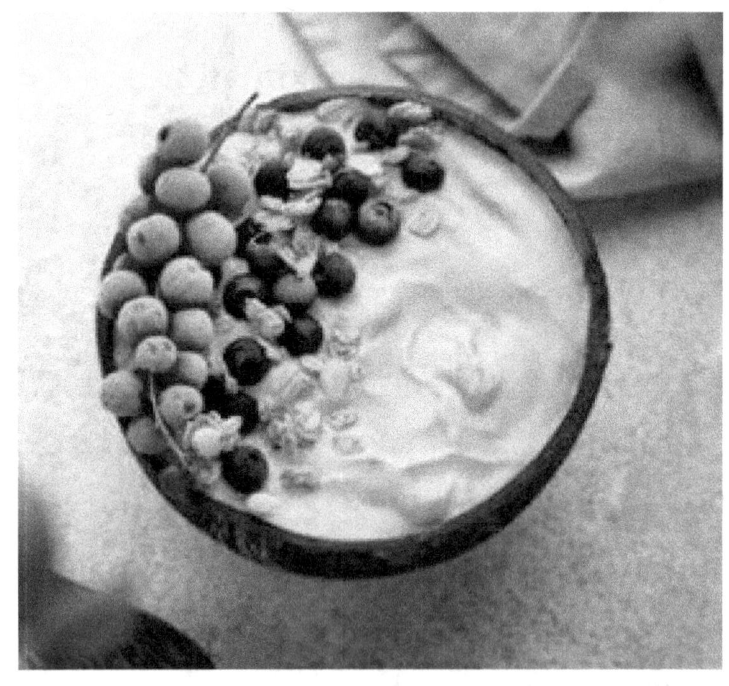

Notes

Your

Observation

Berry Citrus Immunity Booster

Ingredients:

- 1 cup of mixed berries (blueberries, raspberries, strawberries)
- 1/2 cup of orange segments
- 1/2 cup of spinach leaves
- 1 tablespoon of flaxseeds
- 1/2 teaspoon of turmeric powder
- 1/2 cup of coconut water
- Ice cubes (optional)

Instructions:

Get ready the Ingredients:

- Wash the berries and spinach well.
- Peel and segment the orange.
- Measure the flax seeds, turmeric powder, and coconut water.

Combine the ingredients in the blender:

- Combine the mixed berries, orange segments, spinach leaves, flaxseeds, turmeric powder, and coconut water in a blender

Blend until smooth:

- Blend all of the ingredients until the smoothie is smooth and creamy. If required, increase the amount of coconut water.

Ice cubes (optional):

- If you want a cooler smoothie, add a handful of ice cubes and mix until smooth.

Pour and Enjoy Immunity Boost:

- Pour some Berry Citrus Immunity Booster into a glass.
- Sip and enjoy the pleasant taste while reaping the immune-boosting benefits of the berries, citrus, and turmeric.

Nutritional Value Per Serving (Approximate):

Calories: 120 kcal

Protein: 3g

Carbohydrates: 22g

Dietary Fiber: 7g

Sugars: 12g

Fat: 4g

Sodium: 50mg

Potassium: 400mg

Vitamin A: 60% DV

Vitamin C: 120% DV

Calcium: 6% DV

Iron: 2% DV

Notes

Your

Observation

Minty Pineapple Green Smoothie

Ingredients:

- 1 cup of pineapple chunks
- 1/2 cucumber, peeled and sliced
- Handful of fresh mint leaves
- 1/2 lime, juiced
- 1 tablespoon of chia seeds
- 1/2 cup of coconut milk
- Ice cubes (optional)

Instructions:

Get ready the Ingredients:

- Peel and slice the pineapple.
- Peel and slice the cucumber.
- Juice the lime.
- Measure the chia seeds and coconut milk.

Combine the ingredients in the blender:

- Combine the pineapple chunks, cucumber slices, fresh mint leaves, lime juice, chia seeds, and coconut milk in a blender.

Blend until smooth:

- Blend all of the ingredients until the smoothie has a smooth and creamy texture. To alter the thickness, add additional coconut milk as needed.

Ice cubes (optional):

- If you want a cooler smoothie, add a handful of ice cubes and mix until smooth.

Pour and garnish (optional):

- Pour the Minty Pineapple Green Smoothie into a glass.
- Garnish with a sprig of fresh mint for an added kick of flavour.

Sip and Enjoy Tropical Minty Bliss:

- Sip on this delicious smoothie and allow the tropical pineapple, cooling mint, and hydrating cucumber take you to a state of perfect happiness.

Nutritional Value Per Serving (Approximate):

Calories: 150 kcal

Protein: 3g

Carbohydrates: 25g

Dietary Fiber: 6g

Sugars: 15g

Fat: 7g

Sodium: 20mg

Potassium: 400mg

Vitamin A: 10% DV

Vitamin C: 90% DV

Calcium: 8% DV

Iron: 2% DV

Notes

Your

Observation

Chocolate Banana Almond Bliss

Chocolate Banana Almond Bliss

Ingredients:

- 1 banana, frozen
- 2 tablespoons of almond butter
- 1 tablespoon of cacao powder
- 1/2 teaspoon of cinnamon
- 1/2 cup of Greek yogurt (or dairy-free option)
- 1/2 cup of almond milk
- Ice cubes (optional)

Instructions:

Get ready the Ingredients:

- Peel and slice the frozen banana.
- Measure out almond butter, cacao powder, cinnamon, Greek yoghurt, and almond milk.

Combine the ingredients in the blender:

- Combine frozen banana slices, almond butter, cacao powder, cinnamon, Greek yoghurt, and almond milk in a blender.

Blend until creamy:

- Blend all of the ingredients until the smoothie has a creamy, smooth consistency. If required, add extra almond milk.

Ice cubes (optional):

- To increase the coolness factor, add a handful of ice cubes and mix until smooth.

Pour in a glass:

- Pour the Chocolate Banana Almond Bliss smoothie into your glass.

Optional garnish:

- Garnish with cocoa powder or sliced almonds for extra texture.

Sip and Savour the bliss:

- Enjoy the rich and luscious flavours of this chocolatey almond delight, which is a pleasant treat that adheres to lupus-friendly dietary guidelines.

Nutritional Value Per Serving (Approximate):

Calories: 320 kcal

Protein: 12g

Carbohydrates: 30g

Dietary Fiber: 8g

Sugars: 16g

Fat: 18g

Cholesterol: 5mg (when using Greek yogurt)

Sodium: 120mg

Potassium: 600mg

Vitamin A: 2% DV

Vitamin C: 8% DV

Calcium: 25% DV

Iron: 10% DV

Notes

Your

Observation

Ingredients:

- 1 cup of mango chunks (either fresh or frozen)
- 1/2 banana
- 1/2 teaspoon of turmeric powder
- 1 tablespoon of hemp seeds
- 1/2 cup of coconut water
- 1/2 cup of pineapple juice
- Ice cubes (optional)

Instructions:

Get ready the Ingredients:

- If using fresh mango, peel and cut into bits.
- Peel a banana.
- Measure out the turmeric powder, hemp seeds, coconut water, and pineapple juice.

Combine the ingredients in the blender:

- In a blender, combine mango chunks, banana, turmeric powder, hemp seeds, coconut water, and pineapple juice.

Blend until smooth:

- Blend all of the ingredients until the smoothie has a creamy, smooth consistency. If required, increase the amount of coconut water.

Ice cubes (optional):

- For a cool and refreshing experience, add a handful of ice cubes and mix until smooth.

Pour in a glass:

- Pour the Tropical Turmeric Mango Smoothie into a glass.

Garnish (optional):

- To add visual appeal, top with a mango slice or a sprinkling of hemp seeds.

Sip and Enjoy the Tropical Bliss:

- Enjoy the tropical flavours of mango and pineapple while reaping the anti-inflammatory benefits of turmeric. This smoothie is a delicious way to experience the essence of a tropical holiday.

Nutritional Value Per Serving (Approximate):

Calories: 200 kcal

Protein: 4g

Carbohydrates: 35g

Dietary Fiber: 4g

Sugars: 26g

Fat: 7g

Sodium: 30mg

Potassium: 500mg

Vitamin A: 15% DV

Vitamin C: 120% DV

Calcium: 4% DV

Iron: 6% DV

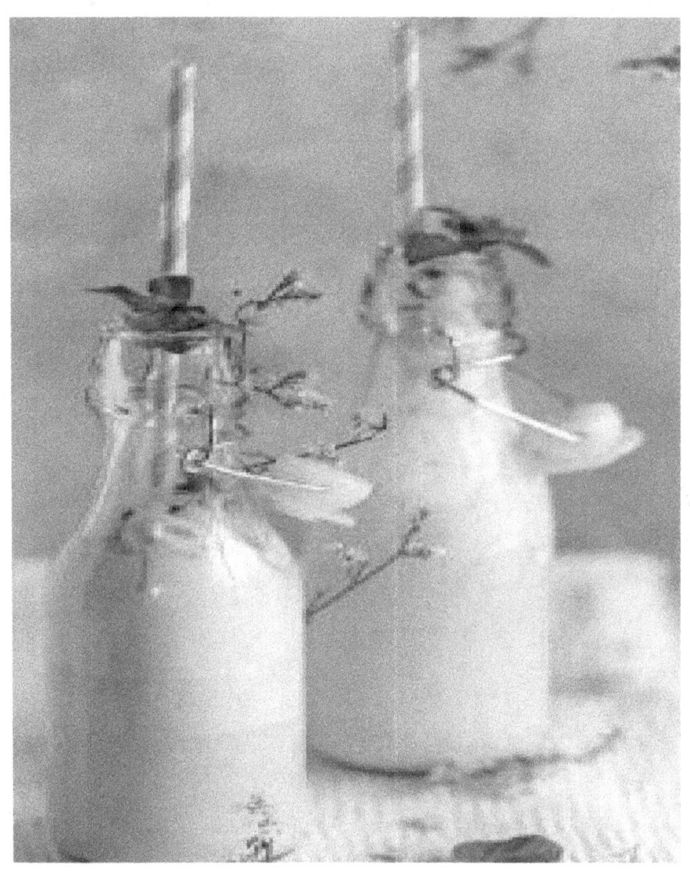

Notes

Your

Observation

Protein-Packed Berry Almond Smoothie

Ingredients:

- 1/2 cup of mixed berries (strawberries, blueberries)
- 1/2 cup of cottage cheese (or tofu for a dairy-free option)
- 1 tablespoon of almond butter
- 1 tablespoon of hemp seeds
- 1/2 cup of almond milk
- Ice cubes (optional)

Instructions:

Assemble the ingredients:

- Wash the berries well.
- Measure out the cottage cheese, almond butter, hemp seeds, and almond milk.

Combine the ingredients in the blender:

- Combine the mixed berries, cottage cheese (or tofu), almond butter, hemp seeds, and almond milk in a blender

Blend until smooth:

- Blend all of the ingredients until the smoothie is creamy and well blended. If required, add additional almond milk to get the desired thickness.

Ice cubes (optional):

- For an additional cold, add a handful of ice cubes and mix until smooth.

Pour in a glass:

- Pour the Protein-Rich Berry Almond Smoothie into a glass.

Optional garnish:

- Add a sprinkling of hemp seeds on top for texture.

Sip and Enjoy the Protein Boost:

- Sip on this delightful smoothie, appreciating the mix of berries, almond butter, and hemp seeds, which add to a protein- and nutrient-rich beverage.

Nutritional Value Per Serving (Approximate):

Calories: 300 kcal

Protein: 18g

Carbohydrates: 20g

Dietary Fiber: 6g

Sugars: 10g

Fat: 16g

Cholesterol: 10mg (if using cottage cheese)

Sodium: 300mg

Potassium: 400mg

Vitamin A: 8% DV

Vitamin C: 30% DV

Calcium: 30% DV

Iron: 10% DV

Notes

Your

Observation

Spinach Blueberry Bliss Smoothie

Ingredients:

- 1 cup of spinach leaves, fresh
- 1/2 cup of blueberries (fresh or frozen)
- 1/2 banana
- 1/2 cup of Greek yogurt (or dairy-free option)
- 1 tablespoon of chia seeds
- 1/2 cup of almond milk
- Ice cubes (optional)

Instructions:

Assemble the Ingredients:

- Wash the spinach leaves well.
- Measure the blueberries, banana, Greek yoghurt, chia seeds, and almond milk.

Combine the ingredients in the blender:

- Combine fresh spinach, blueberries, banana, Greek yoghurt, chia seeds, and almond milk in a blender.

Blend until smooth:

- Blend all of the ingredients until the smoothie is creamy and well-blended. If necessary, add additional almond milk to get the desired thickness.

Ice cubes (optional):

- For an additional cold, add a handful of ice cubes and mix until smooth.

Pour in a glass:

- Pour the Spinach Blueberry Bliss Smoothie into a glass.

Garnish (optional):

- Garnish with a few whole blueberries or chia seeds for a visually pleasing touch.

Sip and Enjoy the Bliss:

Enjoy the refreshing flavour of this nutrient-dense smoothie, which mixes the earthy benefits of spinach with the sweet explosion of blueberries. Sip and enjoy the vivid flavours of health.

Nutritional Value Per Serving (Approximate):

Calories: 180 kcal

Protein: 10g

Carbohydrates: 25g

Dietary Fiber: 6g

Sugars: 12g

Fat: 6g

Cholesterol: 5mg (when using Greek yogurt)

Sodium: 80mg

Potassium: 400mg

Vitamin A: 50% DV

Vitamin C: 30% DV

Calcium: 20% DV

Iron: 2% DV

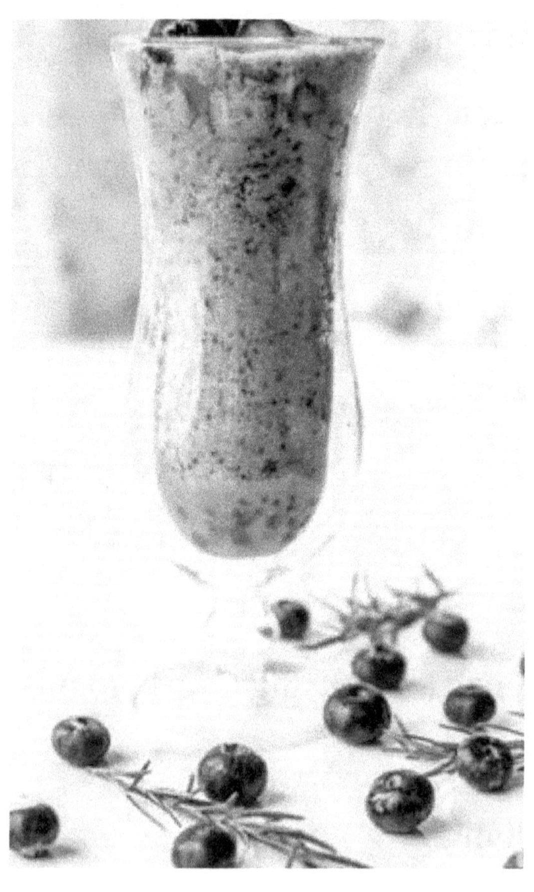

Notes

Your

Observation

Ingredients:

- 1/2 cup of rolled oats (cooked and cooled)
- 1/2 banana
- 1/2 cup of mixed berries (strawberries, blueberries)
- 1/2 cup Greek yogurt (or dairy-free option)
- 1 tablespoon of almond butter
- 1/2 teaspoon of cinnamon
- 1/2 cup of almond milk
- Ice cubes (optional)

Instructions:

Assemble the Oats:

- Cook the rolled oats according to package directions and let it cool before incorporating in the smoothie.

Combine the ingredients in the blender:

- Combine the cooked and cooled muesli, banana, mixed berries, Greek yoghurt, almond butter, cinnamon and almond milk in a blender

Blend until creamy:

- Blend all of the ingredients until the smoothie is creamy and well blended. If required, add additional almond milk to get the desired thickness.

Ice cubes (optional):

- For a cooler, more refreshing texture, add a handful of ice cubes and mix again until smooth.

Pour in a glass:

- Pour the creamy muesli smoothie into a glass.

Optional toppings:

- Garnish with more oats, chopped nuts, or a dab of cinnamon for texture and appearance.

- Enjoy the thick and creamy texture of this oatmeal-infused smoothie. The mix of oats, fruits, and nut butter creates a filling and nutritious snack.

Nutritional Value Per Serving (Approximate):

Calories: 300 kcal

Protein: 15g

Carbohydrates: 40g

Dietary Fiber: 8g

Sugars: 15g

Fat: 10g

Cholesterol: 5mg (when using Greek yogurt)

Sodium: 60mg

Potassium: 450mg

Vitamin A: 10% DV

Vitamin C: 20% DV

Calcium: 25% DV

Iron: 10% DV

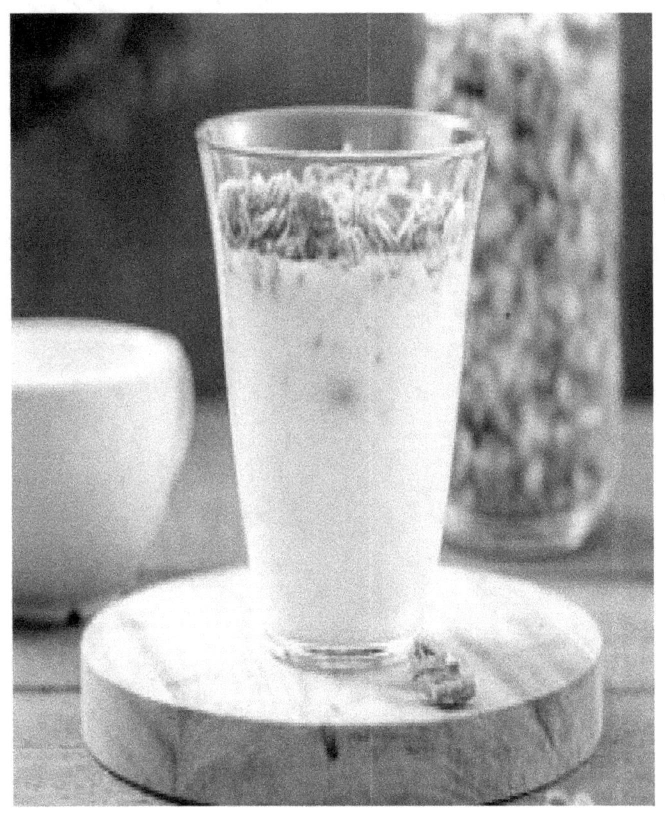

Notes

Your

Observation

Apple cinnamon delight

Ingredients:

- 1 medium-sized apple, cored and chopped
- 1/2 banana
- 1/2 cup of Greek yogurt (or dairy-free option)
- 1/2 teaspoon of ground cinnamon
- 1 tablespoon of almond butter
- 1/2 cup of unsweetened apple juice
- Ice cubes (optional)

Instructions:

Get ready the Ingredients:

- Core and chop the apple.
- Measure the Greek yoghurt, almond butter, and apple juice.

Combine the ingredients in the blender:

- Combine the chopped apples, bananas, Greek yoghurt, ground cinnamon, almond butter, and unsweetened apple juice in a blender

Blend until smooth:

- Blend all of the ingredients until the smoothie is creamy and uniform. If necessary, add additional apple juice to get the desired thickness.

Ice cubes (optional):

- For an additional cold, add a handful of ice cubes and mix until smooth.

Pour in a glass:

- Pour Apple Cinnamon Delight Smoothie into a glass.

Garnish (optional):

- Optionally, sprinkle cinnamon over top for an extra punch of flavour.

Sip & Enjoy the Autumn Vibes:

- With each sip of this smoothie, you will be immersed in the delicious blend of apple and cinnamon. It is the ideal way to enjoy the comforting flavours of autumn while feeding your body with nutritious ingredients.

Nutritional Value Per Serving (Approximate):

Calories: 250 kcal

Protein: 10g

Carbohydrates: 35g

Dietary Fiber: 6g

Sugars: 20g

Fat: 10g

Cholesterol: 5mg (when using Greek yogurt)

Sodium: 30mg

Potassium: 400mg

Vitamin A: 2% DV

Vitamin C: 10% DV

Calcium: 15% DV

Iron: 4% DV

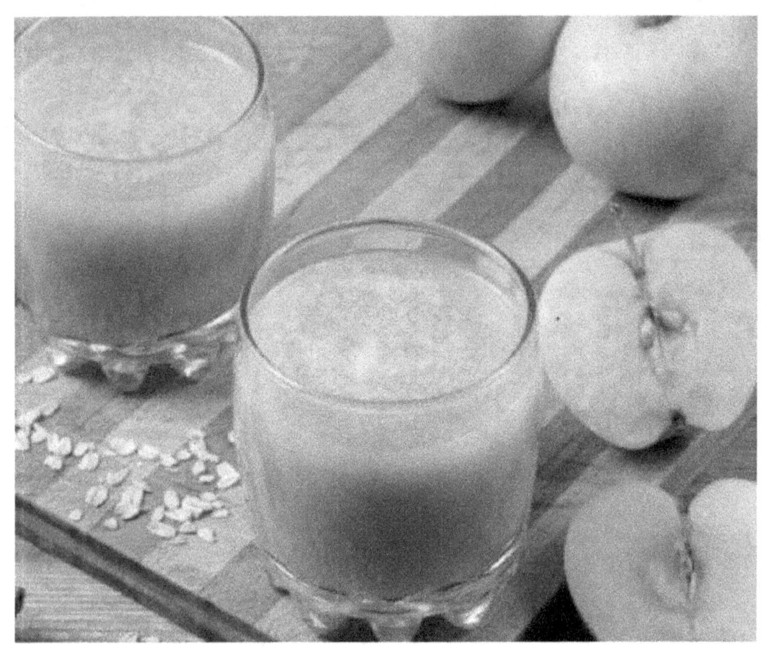

Notes

Your

Observation

Creamy carrot ginger smoothie

Ingredients:

- 1 cup of carrots, peeled and diced
- 1/2 banana
- 1/2 cup Greek yogurt (or dairy-free option)
- 1 tablespoon of fresh ginger, peeled and grated
- 1 tablespoon of honey or maple syrup (optional, for sweetness)
- 1/2 cup of orange juice
- 1/2 cup of almond milk
- Ice cubes (optional)

Instructions:

Get ready the Ingredients:

- Peel and dice carrots.
- Grate some fresh ginger.

Combine the ingredients in the blender:

- Combine the diced carrots, banana, Greek yoghurt, grated ginger, honey or maple syrup (if using), orange juice, and almond milk in a blender.

Blend until smooth:

- Blend all of the ingredients until the smoothie is creamy and uniform. If necessary, add additional almond milk to get the appropriate thickness.

Ice cubes (optional):

- For a colder texture, add a handful of ice cubes and mix until smooth.

Pour in a glass:

- Pour the creamy carrot ginger smoothie into a glass.

Garnish (optional):

- Garnish with a sprinkling of grated ginger or a piece of carrot for added visual appeal.

Sip & Energise:

- With each sip of this smoothie, you will be immersed in the revitalising flavours of carrot and ginger. The mix of sweet carrots and spicy ginger results in a balanced and refreshing beverage to start the day.

Nutritional Value Per Serving (Approximate):

Calories: 200 kcal

Protein: 8g

Carbohydrates: 35g

Dietary Fiber: 5g

Sugars: 20g

Fat: 5g

Cholesterol: 5mg (when using Greek yogurt)

Sodium: 60mg

Potassium: 600mg

Vitamin A: 270% DV

Vitamin C: 90% DV

Calcium: 20% DV

Iron: 2% DV

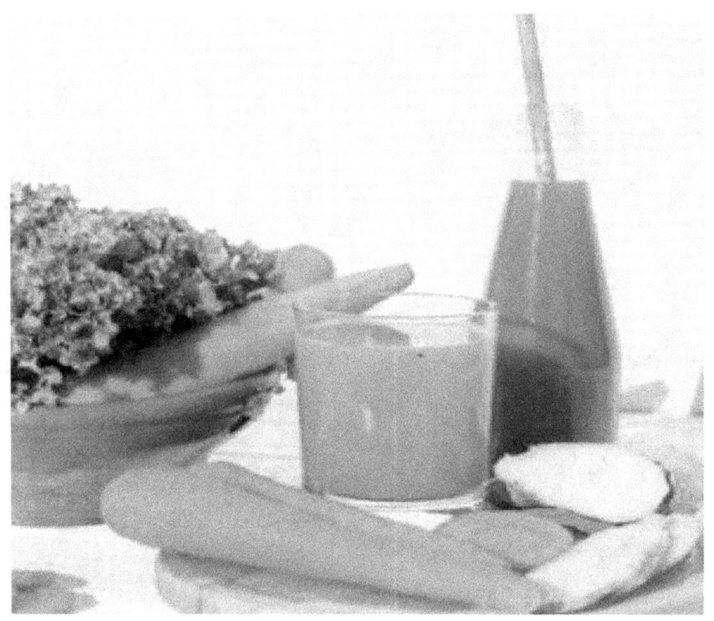

Notes

Your

Observation

Ingredients:

- 1 cup of kale leaves, stems removed
- 1 cup of pineapple chunks (fresh or frozen)
- 1/2 banana
- 1/2 cup of Greek yogurt (or dairy-free option)
- 1 tablespoon of chia seeds
- 1/2 cup of coconut water
- 1/2 cup of water
- Ice cubes (optional)

Instructions:

Get ready the Ingredients:

- Remove the stems from kale leaves.
- Measure the pineapple chunks, banana, Greek yoghurt, and chia seeds.

Combine the ingredients in the blender:

- Combine the kale leaves, pineapple pieces, banana, Greek yoghurt, chia seeds, coconut water, and water in a blender

Blend till refreshingly smooth:

- Blend all of the ingredients until the smoothie has a pleasant, well-blended consistency. If necessary, add additional water to get the desired thickness.

Ice cubes (optional):

- For an additional cold, add a handful of ice cubes and mix until smooth.

Pour in a glass:

- Pour some Kale Pineapple Refresher into a glass.

Garnish (optional):

- Garnish with a piece of pineapple or a sprinkling of chia seeds for decoration.

Sip and Feel the Refreshment:

- With each sip, you will be immersed in the tropical sweetness of kale and pineapple. This smoothie is not only a delicious treat for your taste buds, but it is also a refreshing beverage to get you through the day.

Nutritional Value Per Serving (Approximate):

Calories: 200 kcal

Protein: 10g

Carbohydrates: 35g

Dietary Fiber: 8g

Sugars: 20g

Fat: 5g

Cholesterol: 5mg (when using Greek yogurt)

Sodium: 60mg

Potassium: 600mg

Vitamin A: 150% DV

Vitamin C: 180% DV

Calcium: 20% DV

Iron: 4% DV

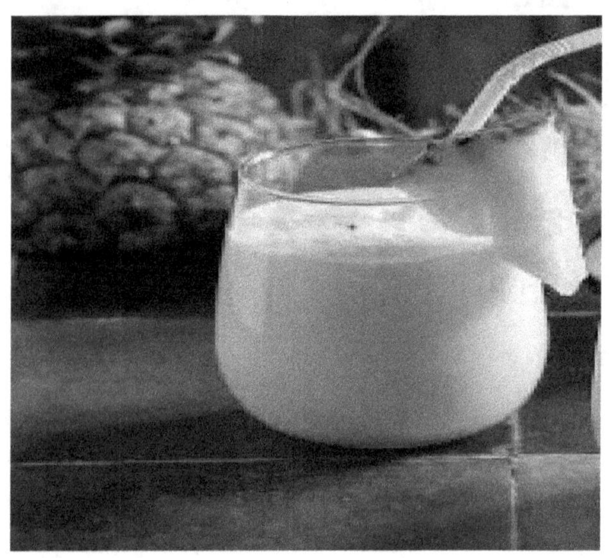

Notes

Your

Observation

Cherry Almond Bliss Smoothie

Ingredients:

- 1 cup of cherries, pitted
- 1/2 banana
- 1/2 cup of Greek yogurt (or dairy-free option)
- 1 tablespoon of almond butter
- 1 tablespoon of flaxseeds
- 1/2 cup of almond milk
- 1/2 cup of water
- Ice cubes (optional)

Instructions:

Get ready the Ingredients:

- Pit the cherries.
- Measure the banana, Greek yoghurt, almond butter, flax seeds, almond milk, and water.

Combine the ingredients in the blender:

- Combine pitted cherries, banana, Greek yoghurt, almond butter, flaxseeds, almond milk, and water in a blender

Blend until blissfully smooth:

- Blend all of the ingredients until the smoothie is perfectly smooth and uniform. If necessary, add additional water to get the required thickness.

Ice cubes (optional):

- For an additional cold, add a handful of ice cubes and mix until smooth.

Pour in a glass:

- Pour Cherry Almond Bliss Smoothie into a glass.

Garnish (optional):

- Garnish with a few whole cherries or a sprinkling of flaxseeds for extra visual appeal.

Sip and enjoy the bliss:

- With each sip, you will be immersed in the delectable blend of cherries and almond. This smoothie strikes the ideal combination of sweetness and nuttiness, providing a delightful and healthy experience.

Nutritional Value Per Serving (Approximate):

Calories: 250 kcal

Protein: 10g

Carbohydrates: 30g

Dietary Fiber: 7g

Sugars: 18g

Fat: 12g

Cholesterol: 5mg (when using Greek yogurt)

Sodium: 60mg

Potassium: 400mg

Vitamin A: 10% DV

Vitamin C: 15% DV

Calcium: 20% DV

Iron: 4% DV

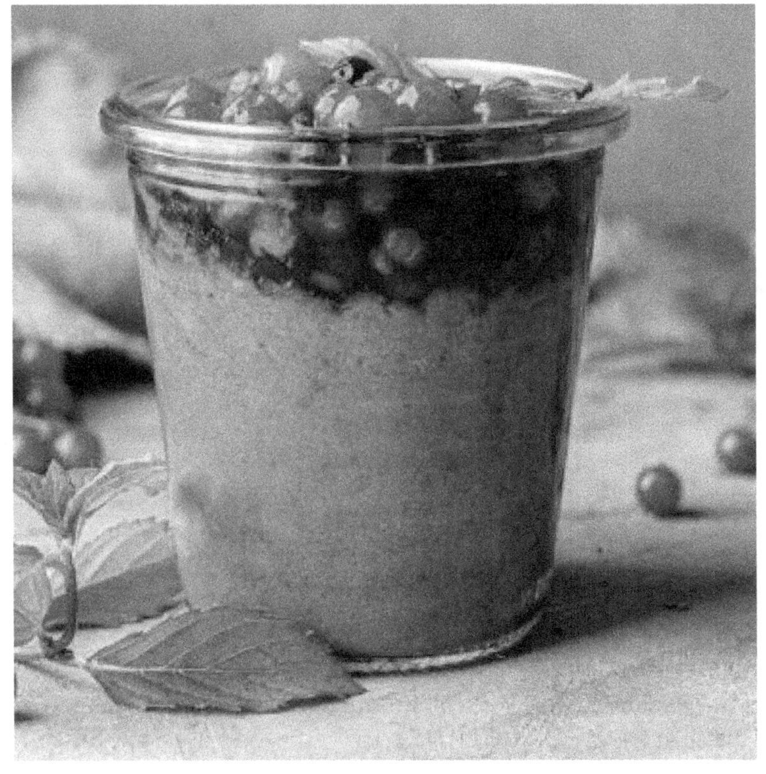

Notes

Your

Observation

Banana walnut smoothie

Ingredients:

- 2 ripe bananas
- 1/4 cup of walnuts
- 1/2 cup of Greek yogurt (or dairy-free option)
- 1 tablespoon of honey or maple syrup (optional, for sweetness)
- 1/2 teaspoon of vanilla extract
- 1/2 cup of milk (dairy or plant-based)
- Ice cubes (optional)

Instructions:

Get ready the Ingredients:

- Peel and slice ripe bananas.
- Measure the walnuts, Greek yoghurt, honey or maple syrup (if using), vanilla essence, and milk.

Combine the ingredients in the blender:

- Combine sliced bananas, walnuts, Greek yoghurt, honey or maple syrup, vanilla extract, and milk in a blender.

Blend until creamy:

- Blend all of the ingredients until the smoothie is creamy and well-blended. If necessary, add additional milk to get the required thickness.

Ice cubes (optional):

- To get a cooler texture, add a handful of ice cubes and mix until smooth.

Pour in a glass:

- Pour Banana Walnut Smoothie into a glass.

Garnish (optional):

- Garnish with crushed walnuts for extra texture.

Sip and enjoy the creaminess:

- With each sip, enjoy the creamy deliciousness of bananas and the crunch of walnuts. This smoothie is not only tasty, but it also provides a delightful method to include healthy fats and natural sweetness into your daily routine.

Nutritional Value Per Serving (Approximate):

Calories: 300 kcal

Protein: 10g

Carbohydrates: 40g

Dietary Fiber: 5g

Sugars: 25g

Fat: 15g

Cholesterol: 5mg (when using Greek yogurt)

Sodium: 40mg

Potassium: 600mg

Vitamin A: 4% DV

Vitamin C: 15% DV

Calcium: 20% DV

Iron: 4% DV

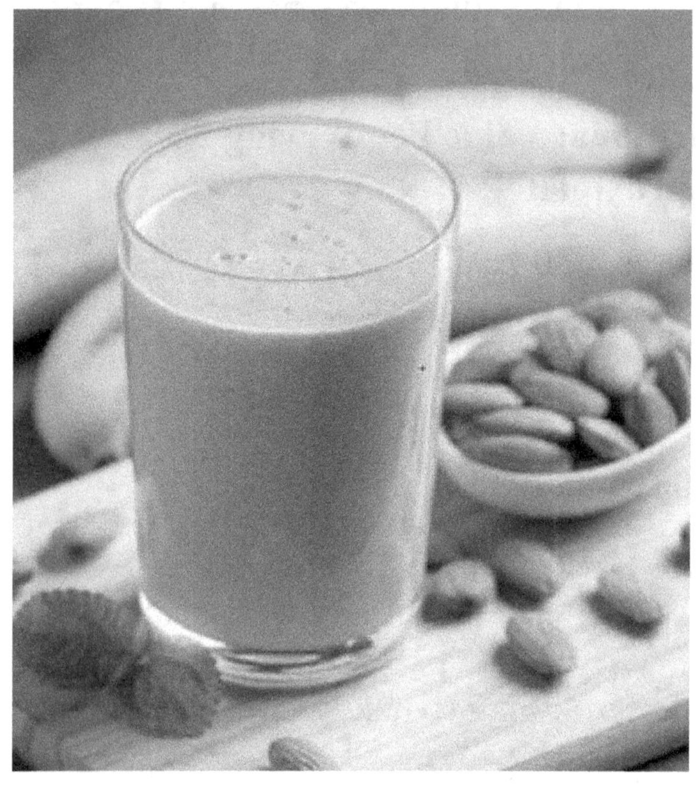

Notes

Your

Observation

Ingredients:

- 1/2 peeled and pitted avocado
- 1 cup of spinach leaves, fresh
- 1/2 banana
- 1/2 cup of Greek yogurt (or dairy-free option)
- 1 tablespoon of chia seeds
- 1 tablespoon of honey or maple syrup (optional, for sweetness)
- 1/2 cup of almond milk
- Ice cubes (optional)

Instructions:

Assemble the Ingredients:

- Peel and pit an avocado.
- Measure fresh spinach leaves, a banana, Greek yoghurt, chia seeds, honey or maple syrup (when in use), and almond milk.

Combine the ingredients in the blender:

- Combine the peeled and pitted avocado, fresh spinach, banana, Greek yoghurt, chia seeds, honey or maple syrup, and almond milk in a blender.

Blend until creamy:

- Blend all of the ingredients until the smoothie is creamy and uniform. If necessary, add additional almond milk to get the desired thickness.

Ice cubes (optional):

- For a cooler, more refreshing texture, add a handful of ice cubes and mix again until smooth.

Pour in a glass:

- Pour the creamy avocado spinach smoothie into a glass.

Garnish (optional):

- Garnish with a few chia seeds or an avocado slice for added visual appeal.

Sip and enjoy the creaminess:

Enjoy the silky texture and refreshing taste of this smoothie. The creamy avocado and nutrient-dense spinach make this a delicious and nutritious beverage.

Nutritional Value Per Serving (Approximate):

Calories: 300 kcal

Protein: 10g

Carbohydrates: 30g

Dietary Fiber: 9g

Sugars: 15g

Fat: 15g

Cholesterol: 5mg (when using Greek yogurt)

Sodium: 40mg

Potassium: 700mg

Vitamin A: 60% DV

Vitamin C: 35% DV

Calcium: 20% DV

Iron: 4% DV

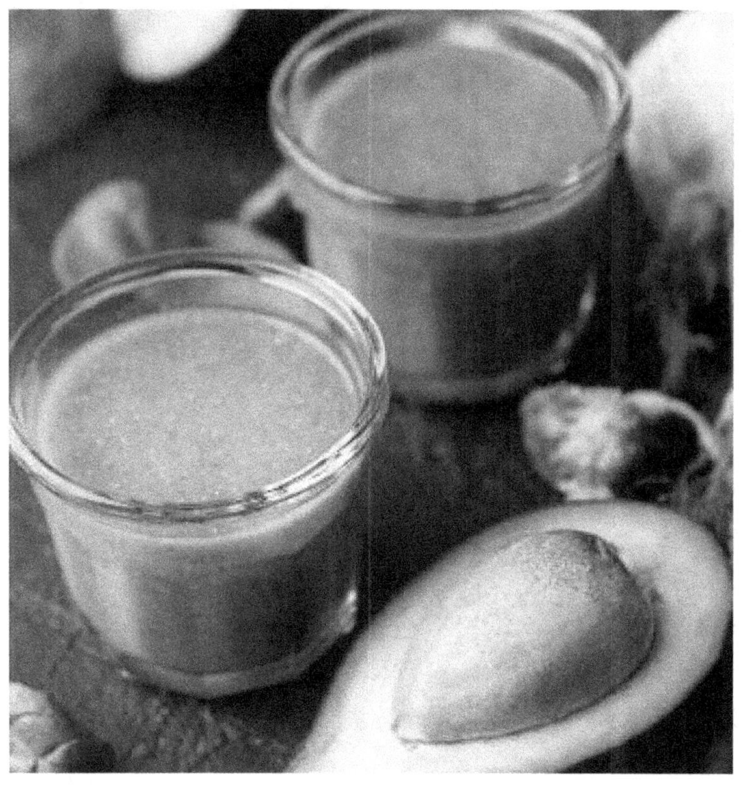

Notes

Your
Observation

CHAPTER 5

Tips for Preparing Lupus-Friendly Smoothies

Creating lupus-friendly smoothies entails taking special dietary precautions and adding ingredients that promote overall health while avoiding possible triggers. Here are specific steps for making lupus-friendly smoothies:

Choose Anti-inflammatory Ingredients:

Prioritise anti-inflammatory substances to help treat lupus symptoms. Include foods that are known to be anti-inflammatory, such as berries, leafy greens, turmeric, ginger, and flax seeds.

Choose Low Glycemic Fruits:

Choose fruits with a low glycemic index to help control your blood sugar levels. Berries, cherries, and apples are excellent options. Limit high-glycemic foods such as watermelon and pineapple.

Incorporate lupus-safe proteins:

Choose lean proteins like Greek yoghurt, tofu, or cottage cheese. These choices deliver protein without increasing inflammation.

Be aware of dairy alternatives:

When choosing dairy replacements, look for ones that are fortified with vitamin D and calcium. Ensure that they are devoid of any ingredients that may cause sensitization.

Include healthy fats:

Include sources of healthy fats such as avocados, chia seeds, flaxseeds, and almond butter. These fats promote satiety and offer important nutrients.

Limit sugar and artificial sweeteners:

Reduce your intake of added sugars and artificial sweeteners, which can cause inflammation. Let the natural sweetness of fruits serve as the major source of sweetness in your smoothies.

Consider omega-3 fatty acids:

Incorporate omega-3 fatty acids from foods such as chia seeds, flaxseeds, and walnuts. These can assist to decrease inflammation and promote overall heart health.

Include leafy greens for nutrients:

Add leafy greens, such as spinach or kale, to boost the nutritional value. These greens are rich in vitamins and minerals yet low in calories.

Be aware of oxalates:

Some lupus patients may be sensitive to the oxalates contained in some greens. If this is a concern, go for low-oxalate greens such as Swiss chard or bok choy.

Hydrate with Lupus-Friendly Liquids:

Use lupus-friendly beverages as a basis, such as coconut water, almond milk, or plain water. These choices provide hydration and may be softer on the digestive tract.

Check for allergies and sensitivities:

Be mindful of any potential dietary allergies or sensitivities linked with lupus. Nightshades (tomatoes, eggplants) and gluten are two common trigger foods.

Consult with healthcare professionals:

Before making substantial dietary changes, speak with healthcare specialists, such as a certified dietitian or a lupus specialist, to verify that your smoothie choices are consistent with your entire treatment plan.

Keep it varied and balanced:

Aim for diversity in your smoothies to guarantee a diverse range of nutrients. Balance macronutrients (carbohydrates, proteins, and fats) to promote overall health.

Monitor Your Body's Response:

Pay attention to how your body reacts to various components. If you have any negative effects, modify your smoothie components appropriately.

Enjoy in moderation:

While smoothies may be a healthy supplement to your diet, consume them in moderation. A varied diet is essential for maintaining overall health.

Using these guidelines, you may make tasty and healthy smoothies that are compatible with a lupus diet. Always prioritise your particular health requirements and seek personalised advice from healthcare specialists.

Fresh vs. Frozen Ingredients

Choosing between fresh and frozen ingredients for your lupus-friendly smoothies depends on a number of circumstances, and both offer advantages. Here's a review of the benefits and downsides of fresh versus frozen ingredients:

Fresh Ingredients:

Benefits:

Nutrient Density: Fresh fruits and vegetables are frequently harvested at their optimal maturity, which maximises nutritious content.

Flavour and Texture: Fresh foods can have a more vivid flavour and a firmer texture, resulting in a more delightful eating experience.

Availability: Seasonal fruits and vegetables are abundantly available and may be sourced locally, which helps regional agriculture.

Drawbacks:

Limited Shelf Life: Fresh products have a limited shelf life, so utilise them quickly to avoid deterioration.

Seasonal Constraints: Some fruits and vegetables are only accessible during specified seasons, restricting diversity.

Frozen Ingredients:

Benefits:

Year-Round Availability: Frozen fruits and veggies are accessible year-round, giving you regular access to a variety of alternatives.

Extended Shelf Life: Frozen products have a longer shelf life than fresh, resulting in reduced food waste.

Convenience: Frozen products require little preparation. They are pre-washed, pre-cut, and ready for usage.

Drawbacks:

Texture Changes: Some fruits, particularly those with a high water content, may alter texture when frozen and thawed.

Potential Nutrient Loss: Although freezing helps to maintain nutrients, there may be some loss during the freezing and thawing process.

Considerations for Lupus Patients:

Nutrient Retention: Both fresh and frozen products can retain critical nutrients, although freezing may result in minimum nutrient deterioration.

Potential allergies: For lupus patients who have allergies or sensitivities, fresh products may be preferable over frozen ones to prevent any additives or processing.

Cost: Frozen fruits and vegetables can be less expensive than fresh food, especially when it is out of season.

Other tips for Making Lupus-Friendly Smoothies:

Mix & Match: Combine fresh and frozen products to balance the benefits of each.

Buy in quantity: Purchase fresh goods in quantity during the season and freeze them for later use.

Check for Additives: When utilising frozen products, look for ones that do not have added sugars or preservatives.

Rotate Varieties: To maintain a diversified and nutrient-dense diet, alternate between fresh and frozen foods.

Ultimately, the decision between fresh and frozen products is based on your own tastes, dietary requirements, and convenience. A mix of the two can give a wide range of nutrients and flavours for lupus-friendly smoothies.

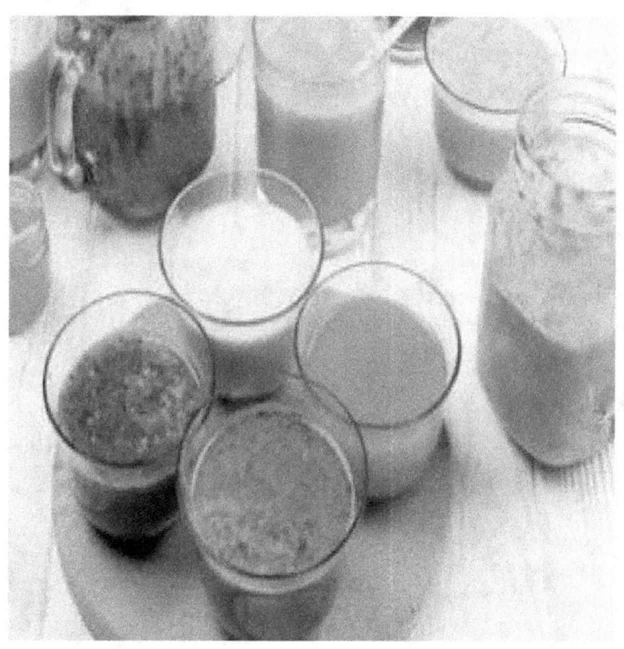

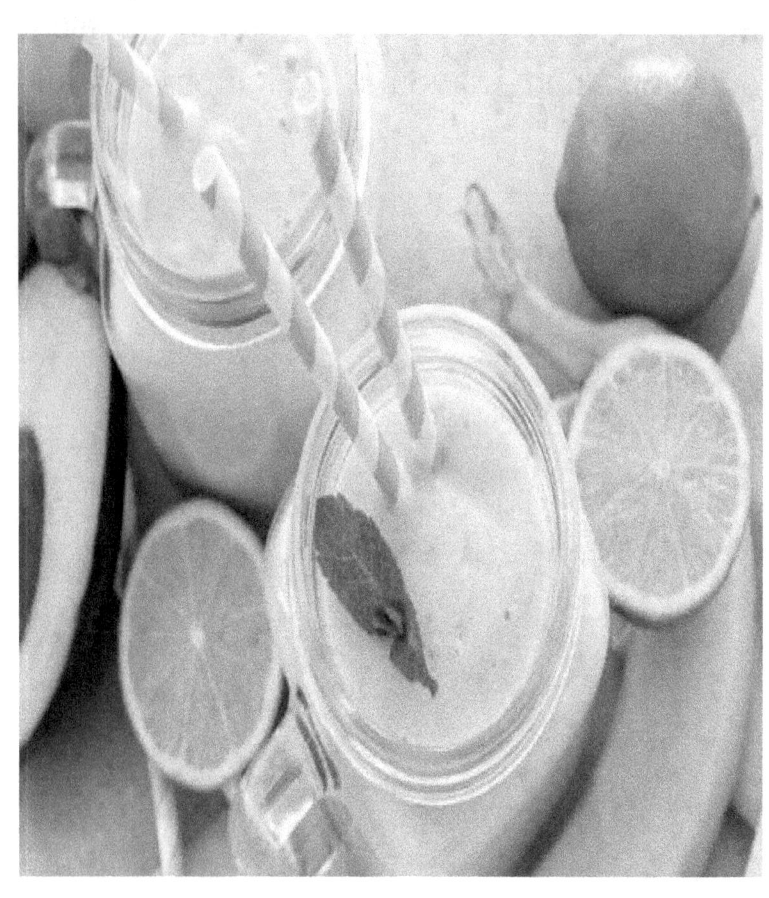

CHAPTER 6: CONCLUSION

Finally, making complete smoothies for lupus requires strategic selections to support overall health. These smoothies can help manage lupus symptoms by combining healthy components such as anti-inflammatory fruits and vegetables with omega-3-rich seeds. Choosing fresh or frozen vegetables, practicing basic cleanliness, and being cognizant of dietary restrictions are all critical for safety. Smoothies may be incorporated into everyday meals, providing a simple and pleasurable approach to increase nutritional consumption. Consult with a healthcare practitioner to ensure that smoothie selections are appropriate for your unique health requirements and lupus management strategy. Lupus-friendly smoothies prioritise balance, diversity, and hydration, making them a delightful and accessible alternative for those managing the challenges of lupus while prioritising their well-being. Enjoying these vivid and nutritious mixes can be a tasty way to promote a balanced and healthful lupus diet.

STAY HEALTHY!